Erick Ramón Silva Bermúdez

HEART DISEASE IN PREGNANCY

Erick Ramón Silva Bermúdez

HEART DISEASE IN PREGNANCY

A brief contextual clinical-epidemiologic analysis

ScienciaScripts

Imprint
Any brand names and product names mentioned in this book are subject to trademark, brand or patent protection and are trademarks or registered trademarks of their respective holders. The use of brand names, product names, common names, trade names, product descriptions etc. even without a particular marking in this work is in no way to be construed to mean that such names may be regarded as unrestricted in respect of trademark and brand protection legislation and could thus be used by anyone.

Cover image: www.ingimage.com

This book is a translation from the original published under ISBN 978-613-9-43990-4.

Publisher:
Sciencia Scripts
is a trademark of
Dodo Books Indian Ocean Ltd. and OmniScriptum S.R.L publishing group

120 High Road, East Finchley, London, N2 9ED, United Kingdom
Str. Armeneasca 28/1, office 1, Chisinau MD-2012, Republic of Moldova, Europe
Printed at: see last page
ISBN: 978-620-8-17739-3

CLINICAL-EPIDEMIOLOGICAL CHARACTERISATION OF HEART DISEASE IN PREGNANCY

ERICK RAMÓN SILVA BERMÚDEZ

2024

THOUGHT

Before all human suffering, as far as you can: devote yourself not only to alleviating it without delay but also to destroying its causes; devote yourself not only to destroying its causes but also to alleviating it. without delay.

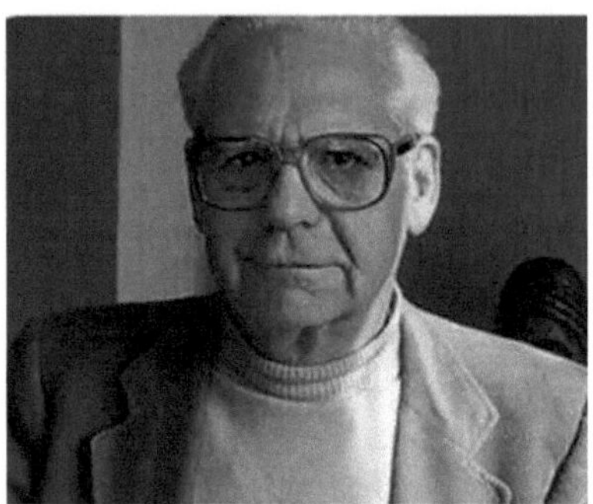

Michel Quoist (1921-1997)

DEDICATION

To my family and friends: Inexhaustible source of my dedication.

ACKNOWLEDGEMENTS

I am deeply grateful to all my teachers and colleagues for providing me with the necessary knowledge throughout my training, especially to the teachers of the Cardiology Service of the Vladimir Ilyich Lenin Hospital who, apart from being my teachers, were also my co-workers and family during the residency.
To Dr. Edel Lachataignerais Popa who, as my tutor, was able to offer me all his valuable assistance and collaboration in the development of this research.
My eternal gratitude to Dr. Fabián Ignacio Fernández Chelada and Dr. Bernardo Enrique Fernández Chelada for their unconditional help in my life and development of my work.

Gratitude to DrC. Carlos Viltre Calderón for drawing the curtain on the publication for me. science. Thank you all.

INDEX

SUMMARY

This book is the result of a research presented in option to the title of first degree specialist in cardiology. The descriptive observational study was carried out at the General University Hospital "Vladimir Ilich Lenin" in Holguin, Cuba, from January to December 2022. The general objective of the thesis was to contribute to the Mother and Child Programme, to a better understanding of the evolution of pregnancy in patients with heart disease, through the description of a sample of this condition. The universe was made up of 60 pregnant women with heart disease who were seen at the heart disease and pregnancy clinic. The cases were followed up and the primary information was collected directly from each patient by the author of the study through a survey prepared in accordance with the proposed objectives, and the information obtained was contrasted with the data in the medical records. For the processing of the information, a database was created to allow statistical processing and the analysis and discussion of the results. The results of the study showed that 31.7% of the cases had congenital heart disease, with bicuspid aorta being the most frequent. In the group of other causes, mitral valve prolapse predominated. Thirty percent of the patients under study had rheumatic heart disease, with mitral stenosis and mitral valve insufficiency being the most frequent. In 85% of the pregnant women, the heart diseases were diagnosed before pregnancy. The cardiologist advised 93.3% of the pregnant women that they could continue the pregnancy. The maternal complications secondary to heart disease were minimal and occurred in the third trimester. 65% delivered euthanically with a prematurity index of 3.3%; no perinatal or maternal mortality was reported.

INTRODUCTION

The adult survival of patients with heart disease has increased as a result of advances in cardiovascular surgery and new technologies, resulting in a new and growing population of patients of childbearing age with operated heart disease.

It is now recognised that pregnancy can coexist with heart disease and while it is the leading cause of non-obstetric maternal morbidity and mortality, it is possible to achieve a successful pregnancy if there is adequate counselling in assessing the risks, including biological, psychological and socio-economic risks.

The foetal risks and teratogenicity of proposed treatments, such as the use of anticoagulants and certain specific transient or permanent contraceptive actions, are also important. Rational use of contraceptive methods is essential for the reproductive health of women with heart disease.

The presence of pregnancy-associated heart disease is a serious problem because, although the incidence ranges from 0.4-2%, for many it is the leading cause of non-obstetric maternal mortality, and its incidence is increasing because of developments in cardiology and cardiovascular surgery that have allowed women with congenital and other heart diseases not only to survive but also to have a successful pregnancy.

The decrease in the frequency of rheumatic fever and thus of possible residual heart disease, as well as the improved medical-surgical treatment of congenital heart disease, mean that the obstetrician is faced with problems that differ greatly from those of two or three decades ago. The 20:1 ratio of rheumatic to congenital heart disease is now 2:1 in many hospitals.

The remaining heart-related diseases are a less frequent group and include arterial hypertension, ischaemic heart disease and arrhythmias. Pregnancies in mothers with heart disease have also been associated with a higher incidence of preterm birth, intrauterine growth retardation, foetal distress and a perinatal mortality of about 18%, ten times higher than the general mortality rate. In congenital heart disease (CHD), the association of hereditary risk must also be assessed.

Gestation imposes a considerable haemodynamic overload on the maternal cardiocirculatory system, such that it can produce semiological manifestations that in a normal state simulate heart disease. The diseased heart is able to cope with this overload in general, in The quality of life of the mother and maternal and foetal morbidity and mortality will depend to a large extent on this.

In the pregnant woman with heart disease, the lives of both mother and foetus are at stake; the maternal cardiac reserve is limited by the existing heart disease, and requires it to cope with the additional circulatory demands of pregnancy. This in turn affects the maternal cardiovascular system and maternal heart disease can affect either the pregnant mother or the foetus.

Authors such as Bouzas and Gatzoulis (2005) state that pregnant women with cyanotic congenital heart disease or pulmonary hypertension have an increased risk of complications and maternal and foetal mortality, so pregnancy is not advisable in these patients; on the other hand, most patients with acyanotic congenital heart disease tolerate pregnancy without complications and mortality is the same as in patients without heart disease.

Myometrial lesions represent 90% of the observations, with an overwhelming predominance of stenosis and rheumatic aetiology; congenital conditions are reported at 6%, other cardiac conditions reach up to 4%, although a remarkable modification in the type of heart diseases found has been reported in the last decades, when the incidence of conditions of rheumatic origin is reduced; this circumstance has resulted in a change in their relative incidence during gestation, which now show a mathematical ratio of 3:1.

Congenital heart diseases are accepted with a constant "natural" frequency of 0.8 per 100 live births and also, among other things, because of the efficiency and effectiveness of current therapy for rheumatic diseases. The rate of caesarean section increases in relation to the functional degree of these patients, it is between 10 to 20 %.

In Cuba in the last 30 years the frequency of congenital and rheumatic heart disease has decreased by almost 50 %, which shows a change in the type of heart disease, according to Mendoza-Calderón et al (2012).

As medical and surgical treatment of congenital heart disease improves, the specialist caring for pregnant women faces a spectrum that differs greatly from that of two or three decades ago.

A similar incidence is reported in the West, where mitral valve prolapse predominates. The remarkable progress that cardiovascular surgery has achieved at this time has produced another important change, we now see an increasing number of pregnant women undergoing corrective or palliative cardiovascular operations that allow them to successfully fulfil their desire to procreate. Many concepts have changed on this subject and in consultation, comprehensive, multidisciplinary, highly specialised care in pre- and post-conception life has also reached cardiac patients. For these reasons, the assessment of this type of patient is becoming increasingly necessary, which makes it possible to define the most suitable time for gestation and must include an analysis of the resources required to meet their needs, with respect for the criteria of evidence-based medicine and the use of a multidisciplinary approach.

Activities are implemented in primary, secondary and tertiary care, with the basic principle that it is preferable to diagnose and treat heart disease before pregnancy. Therefore the prognosis of this type of pregnancy depends on: cardiac functional capacity, complications that increase the cardiac load, associated diseases such as hypertension (HTN), quality of medical services and socio-economic factors. In Holguín province, in the north-eastern part of Cuba, the incidence of heart disease is low in relation to the total number of patients attended in the provincial maternity ward. In general terms, the prognosis of pregnancy in patients with heart disease depends on the severity of the heart disease and the overall cardiac functional work, as expressed in the New York Heart Association classification of functional capacity grades I, II, III and IV. Patients in groups III and IV are at the highest risk.

It is common to see patients with uncomplicated heart disease or with functional capacity grade I and II, who have been advised to avoid or interrupt pregnancy and on many occasions discrepancies are created in them and their relatives. The prohibition of pregnancy for all patients with heart disease should be made after a comprehensive team assessment. Pregnancy termination as a means of preserving or restoring cardiac compensation is rarely necessary.

The aforementioned problems motivated us to programme a follow-up of heart patients during the course of pregnancy and childbirth with clinical-epidemiological assessment of their behaviour and to propose appropriate guidance for heart patients in the fertile stage and to detect their risk factors. This work, together with the experiences acquired by the author, will facilitate the creation of a single criterion in the collective that will allow the provision of adequate obstetric advice to these patients, contributing at the same time to the Mother and Child Programme that is managed in the province by the "Vladimir Ilich Lenin" General University Hospital. Bearing in mind that research on the subject is scarce, and that there are no statistical records showing exact data, the research problem posed is: How does heart disease behave clinically and epidemiologically in pregnant women in the Hospital General Universitario "Vladimir Ilich Lenin" in the city of Holguín, during the period from January to December 2022?

OBJECTIVES

General:

To determine the clinical-epidemiological characteristics of heart disease in pregnant women.

Specific:

- Identify the main heart diseases associated with pregnancy.
- To determine the time of diagnosis of heart disease according to pregnancy and the orientation received in obstetric counselling.
- Group patients according to New York Heart Association functional class.
- Determine the complications that occurred and the period of pregnancy in which they occurred.
- To determine the relationship between cardiac complications and functional physical capacity.
- Identify the final route of delivery and perinatal morbidity and mortality.

THEORETICAL FRAMEWORK

Pregnancy and the peripartum period bring with them significant cardiocirculatory changes that cause real stress, to which a pregnant woman with normal cardiac function adapts physiologically, but when there is underlying heart disease, pregnancy becomes a dangerous phenomenon with rapid clinical and haemodynamic deterioration, which can decompensate the patient, increase the risk of maternal-fetal complications and eventually cause death.

Pregnancy by itself could cause heart failure in a cardiac patient in whom there were no signs of heart failure at the beginning of pregnancy, and in whom, in the absence of pregnancy, the cardiac lesion by itself would not have led to heart failure in such a short period of time.

Generally speaking, pregnancy is one of the most important stages for women. It is the materialisation of a couple's well-being, the consolidation of a relationship, and the continuation of life. During pregnancy, a series of physiological changes occur in all organs and systems to meet the metabolic demands of the growing foetus.

These changes are very important, particularly on the cardiovascular system in female heart disease survivors. The entire cardiovascular physiology changes abruptly to adapt to the new metabolic demands. And these changes increase the risk of cardiovascular complications and decompensation during pregnancy and labour in women with heart disease.

Globally, it is known that, of all pregnancies, between 1 and 4% are affected by different cardiovascular diseases, such as arterial hypertension, heart failure, valvular diseases, arrhythmias, among others. But pregnancies specifically affected by congenital heart disease deserve special attention.

Women with heart disease were for many years "condemned" to be unable to bear children because of the increased risk of maternal mortality that pregnancy posed to them, hence marriage, pregnancy and breastfeeding were practically limited for these patients.

There are authors (Gutiérrez Aliaga, et. al., (2011) & Labrada Comas, et. al., (2016) who state that many therapeutic errors have been and are made, and that the aphorism that says: "In case of heart disease it would be preferable that the woman does not marry, that if she marries she does not become a mother, that if she has been a mother unwisely once or twice, she does not become one in the future, that in case of a happy birth she refrains from breastfeeding her child" is inaccurate. In the middle of the last century, more than 90% of children born with complex congenital heart disease (CHD) died before adulthood; today, thanks to advances in the field of cardiovascular surgery and perinatal intensive care and the impact of pregnancy on pregnant women diagnosed with congenital heart disease this is not the case (Hall, et. al., 2011), 2011) In 1930 it was estimated that about 1-2% of pregnancies were complicated by maternal heart disease and that 6% of women died during pregnancy. (Casellas, 2011).

In a study of maternal deaths in the UK (1997-1999), heart disease equalled thromboembolism as the leading cause. Thirty percent of cardiac deaths were due to congenital heart disease, 15% to ischaemic heart disease and the remainder to other acquired heart disease.

The association between pregnancy and pre-existing or onset of heart disease during pregnancy is the leading cause of indirect maternal death. This is due to the fact that 85% of paediatric patients with congenital heart disease survive to adulthood, thus increasing the incidence of pregnancies complicated by cardiovascular disease, as well as to the increasing age of primigravidae ranging from 28.8 to 31.2 years.

In Western studies, congenital heart disease accounts for 75-82% of heart disease in pregnancy, while in non-Western countries, rheumatic valve disease is the main cause.

The ROPAC registry (Registry of Pregnancy And Cardiac Disease), the most important registry in relation to cardiovascular disease and pregnancy, has shown that the most prevalent cardiovascular disease in developed countries is CHD in 70% of cases, compared to valve disease in 55% of cases in developing countries.

In relation to the population of Latin America (LATAM) and the Caribbean, we know today an estimated number of CCAs of more than 1.8 million in South America and 657,000 in Central America and the Caribbean, of which at least 50% are women of childbearing age. This population will have an annual growth of 5-6%, so it is to be expected that the number of pregnancies with heart disease will also increase.

Based on the knowledge of the more than 1.8 million CCAs living in South America and the 657,000 in Central America and the Caribbean, we can estimate that at least 1.2 million women of childbearing age have heart disease. Since the past decades, a change in the type of maternal heart disease has been observed, with a gradual increase in the number of mothers with congenital heart disease and a decrease in those with rheumatic heart disease, reflecting a sharp decline in the incidence of fever. rheumatic diseases and much better medical and surgical treatment of congenital heart disease, allowing many girls not only to reach reproductive age, but to do so in a condition that allows pregnancy (Aguilera Castro, et. al., 2011).

The World Health Organisation (WHO) considers four groups: group I, no increase in morbidity and mortality during pregnancy for concomitant heart disease; group II, small increase in mortality and moderate increase in morbidity; group III, with a significant increase in mortality and morbidity, the patient requires multidisciplinary advice and, if she decides to become pregnant, management in a referral unit; group IV, includes heart disease and extreme risk situations with high mortality, for which pregnancy is contraindicated, and if it has occurred, voluntary termination should be considered.

The classification of congenital and acquired heart disease according to this risk scale empowers the cardiologist with no experience with pregnant women to make a decision that will allow for the prompt referral of high-risk patients to a multidisciplinary team (Reinoso, et. al., 2012).

The situation of women in our society has changed dramatically and has led to a shift in time and in the priority of gestational desire, which places them in situations of greater risk for themselves and their future infants. Similarly, advances in cardiology and paediatric cardiovascular surgery have made it possible to modify the natural history of congenital heart disease and the daily lives of patients with these conditions (Vega Gutiérrez, et. al., 2012).

General overview of heart disease in pregnancy.

Signs of heart disease in pregnant women

- Cyanosis
- Digital hypocracy
- Persistent jugular ingurgitation
- Systolic murmur greater than III-IV/VI
- Diastolic murmur
- Cardiomegaly
- Documented sustained arrhythmia

▪ Fixed splitting of the second noise

▪ Signs of pulmonary hypertension

▪ Bibasal crackles.

Symptoms of heart disease in pregnant women

▪ Progressive dyspnoea

▪ Orthopnoea

▪ Paroxysmal nocturnal dyspnoea

▪ Haemoptysis

▪ Exertional syncope

▪ Exertional angina

Cardiovascular physiology in normal pregnancy

Knowledge of the haemodynamic changes that occur during normal pregnancy is very important in the management of the patient with cardiovascular disease. Cardiovascular adaptations in pregnancy are intended to increase uterine perfusion to meet the demands of the growing foeto-placental unit. Maternal blood volume begins to rise at six weeks gestation; there is a rapid increase until around 32 weeks and reaches a plateau thereafter, at a maximum increase of 50% above non-pregnant.

Although red blood cell mass and plasma volume are increased, there is a relative increase in plasma volume compared to red blood cell mass, causing the 'physiological anaemia of pregnancy'. The increase in blood volume is partly related to the oestrogen-induced increase in plasma renin. In pregnancy, renin is not only produced in the kidneys, but also in the uterus and liver (Valladares-Carvajal, et al., 2011).

Physiological changes during pregnancy and childbirth

Major physiological changes that occur during pregnancy and childbirth include the following:

▪ Progressive increase in plasma volume (up to 30-50%), especially from the 2nd trimester onwards. This is due to relaxation of the vascular smooth muscles by endothelial factors (prostacyclin and oestrogens) and hydrosaline retention.

▪ 10-15% increase in heart rate.

- Cardiac output (CO) increases to 30-50% at around 24-26 weeks gestation, and then remains stable.
- Reduction of peripheral vascular resistance leading to a decrease in systemic blood pressure (T.A.).
- Hypercoagulable state that increases the risk of thromboembolism.
- During labour there is an increase in C.G. and A.T. with uterine contractions. Immediately after delivery there is an abrupt increase in preload due to uterine contractions. decompression of the inferior vena cava and the return of uterine blood to the systemic circulation.
- The cardiovascular adaptations associated with gestation return approximately 6 weeks after delivery.

In general, the physiological changes that occur in all organs and systems during pregnancy are intended to allow the woman to adapt to the new conditions necessary to respond to the metabolic demands of the growing foetus. The changes in the cardiovascular system during pregnancy represent one of the most significant, and with regard to congenital cardiovascular diseases they are of great relevance; as they predict from very early stages the success or failure of the pregnancy.

The function of these changes is to respond to the haemodynamic demands of volume that must go to the enlarged uterus due to gestation and its secondarily hypertrophied vascular system. This increases the supply of nutrients and trace elements for foetal and placental growth. The increase in circulating volume attenuates the impact of the fall in venous return (secondary to the fall in systemic vascular resistance and the mechanical effect of the uterus on systemic venous return). And finally, it protects the mother at the time of bleeding associated with childbirth.

As soon as circulatory volume increases, cardiac output (CO) increases from 5-8 weeks of gestation. These changes continue to increase by 50% between 16 and 20 weeks of gestation, resulting in a volume of 4.6 l/min to 8.7 l/min. Blood flow is redistributed, with 25% of the GCS reaching the pregnant uterus and placenta; flow to the skin, kidneys and mammary glands also increases significantly. The increase in GCS may increase by a further 20% in multiple gestations.In response to this increase in volume, the ventricles dilate and accommodate the new circulatory volume. But this does not translate into a net increase in end-diastolic pressures. The end-diastolic volume of the left ventricle (LV) increases, but the end-systolic volume remains the same, resulting in a pure increase in ejection fraction. During this volume expansion, not only the circulating volume expressed as plasma volume increases, but also the number of red blood cells; but comparatively more plasma volume increases, resulting in dilutional anaemia. The LV develops a slight physiological hypertrophy, with an increase in mass of 30-35%, and reverses within the first 3 months postpartum. LV diastolic function does not change with pregnancy. Due to the increased abdominal and pelvic pressures caused by the enlarged uterus, systemic venous return from the lower limbs is reduced and slowed, which secondarily causes oedema of the lower limbs and pelvic area, predisposing to deep vein thrombosis (associated with other risk factors).The pressure in the inferior vena cava and femoral veins increases by up to 75%. And due to the collateral circulation the venous return is maintained, thus ensuring a stable filling pressure. Systolic, diastolic and mean blood pressure fall to values about half pregestational, with the fall in diastolic pressure being more marked, caused by the neurohormonal effects of progestogens with reduced systemic vascular resistance (SVR), which gradually decreases, peaking at 20 weeks (up to 35% lower than pregestational values). It then increases as gestation reaches term; however, it remains approximately 20% below baseline, and this decrease in blood pressure may remain after delivery as long-term vascular changes are possible. Pulmonary capillary wedge pressure and central venous pressure do not change significantly. At term there may be an increase in brachial systolic blood pressure, secondary to increased RSV due to aortic compression. 10-15% of pregnant women present with supine hypotension syndrome which manifests with bradycardia plus hypotension, resulting from a significant drop in venous return which cannot be adequately compensated by the cardiovascular system.

Changes resulting from physical examinations on the cardiovascular system

Generally speaking, pregnancy causes an increase in cardiac size due to an increase in the volume and force of contraction. In addition to this, the elevation of the diaphragm due to the enlarged uterus causes changes in the physical examination which we will describe below: on auscultation the first heart sound may be accentuated, with mitral and tricuspid component splitting; the second heart sound has little change and varies less with respiration; a third and fourth heart sound may be auscultated in up to 16% of pregnant women and usually disappears at term; in some patients murmurs appear, usually grade II systolic audible at the left sternal border, due to the aforementioned volume changes causing dilatation of the tricuspid annulus.Diaphragmatic displacement causes movement of the heart to the left and cephalad, resulting in a displacement of the point of maximal impulse in the same direction and a larger visualisation of the cardiac silhouette on the chest X-ray. Elevation of the diaphragm generates movement of the heart, resulting in a larger cardiac silhouette on the chest X-ray.The electrocardiogram also has changes that are more marked in the third trimester. Increased heart rate, shortened PR and QT segments, QRS axis shifts to the right in the first trimester but may shift to the left in the third trimester. A depressed or flattened ST segment may also be seen in the left precordial and limb leads. Occasionally inverted T waves may also be found in leads DIII, V1-V3.Echocardiographic study shows eccentric left ventricular hypertrophy from 12 weeks with a 50% increase in mass at term. The diameters of the valve annuli increase and some degree of regurgitation can be seen, but the aortic annulus remains unchanged.

Maternal risk

Risk stratification is based on basic knowledge about physiological changes during pregnancy, on established knowledge of certain conditions involving high mortality. Recently, a couple of prospective observational studies on risk factors for cardiovascular complications during pregnancy have been published, as well as small disease-specific studies, mostly retrospective and without echocardiographic information. In general, the issues to be considered are:

- Diseases involving limited cardiac output, i.e. left-sided obstructive conditions, will not be well tolerated.
- Falling peripheral vascular resistances will mean that left-sided valvular insufficiencies and left-right shunts will be well tolerated, whereas, for the same reason, conditions with right-left shunts will not be well tolerated.
- It is well established that primary pulmonary hypertension and Eisenmenger's syndrome carry a prohibitive risk, with 30-50% mortality during pregnancy.
- The need for anticoagulation secondary to mechanical prostheses implies a significant maternal and foetal risk.

The risk to the foetus

Congenital heart disease is the most common group of congenital anomalies and has a high morbidity and mortality. The current approach in foetal medicine is to approach the foetus as a patient.

Prenatal diagnosis of congenital heart disease should be performed as part of the fetal anatomical assessment in each trimester of pregnancy. Such assessment is indicated for all pregnant women, since most congenital heart disease occurs in the low-risk population, i.e. without identifiable risk factors.There is a small group of heart diseases that, due to their developmental nature and pathophysiology, can only be identified late in pregnancy or even after birth. These include coarctation of the aorta, tetralogy of Fallot, septal defects and cardiac tumours.As pregnancy progresses, factors such as fetal position, fetal movements, ossification of the ribs, amount of amniotic fluid, etc., make assessment more difficult. Fetal Doppler echocardiography is a detailed assessment to identify and characterise pre-birth fetal cardiac abnormalities. The evaluation includes axial and complementary ultrasound slices; assessment of cardiac function and rhythm, and cardiac biometry.

It allows the identification of foetuses requiring immediate pre- and post-natal interventions. In at-risk patients, assessment should be performed in each trimester. After the diagnosis of congenital heart disease, management should be carried out by a multidisciplinary team made up of different specialists: paediatric cardiologist, obstetrician, perinatal geneticist, neonatologist, psychologist, foetal surgeon and paediatric surgeon according to the needs of each particular case. In this way it is possible to establish the optimal time of birth, the appropriate site and postnatal management, according to the therapeutic options available and the perinatal prognosis. The main objectives are to provide an accurate diagnosis, to provide clear prognostic information, to offer treatment options and to help parents to make decisions while respecting their autonomy.

The diagnosis of critical congenital heart disease allows for the coordination of scheduled birth and a reduction in mortality prior to surgery, compared to postnatal diagnosis. In foetuses with selected pathology, foetal therapy can modify the natural history of the disease and thus improve its prognosis, such as transplacental administration of antiarrhythmic drugs in fetuses with arrhythmias and the risk of heart failure, balloon aortic valvuloplasty in fetuses with critical aortic stenosis, balloon pulmonary valvuloplasty in fetuses with pulmonary atresia, and atrioseptostomy in patients with hypoplastic left ventricle.

The risk of transmission of congenital heart disease to offspring should be considered before conception. In general, this risk can be estimated at around 4%, while the risk of congenital heart disease in the general population is 0.8%.

Some conditions are inherited in an autosomal dominant pattern, such as DiGeorge syndrome, Marfan syndrome, hypertrophic cardiomyopathy or Noonan syndrome, with a 50% risk of transmission. In these cases, the future possibility of performing a chorionic biopsy at 12 weeks of pregnancy will allow prenatal diagnosis.The incidence of foetal and neonatal complications in pregnant women with heart disease is higher than in the general population, and intrauterine growth retardation, prematurity, intracranial haemorrhage and foetal loss are the main complications reported.

Treatment of heart disease during pregnancy

Many women with heart disease around the world have had inadequate pregnancies, but few of them have been assessed and monitored by appropriate medical groups (cardiologist, internist, obstetrician, geneticist, neonatologist and anaesthesiologist). Therefore, according to their baseline conditions and gestational status, it is important for patients to recognise normal and abnormal symptoms in order to be consulted in a timely manner and treated by an appropriate medical team. Advances in cardiac surgery have changed the history of congenital heart disease, allowing an increasing number of women to reach adulthood and be able to carry a pregnancy. Only in developing countries, where rheumatic heart disease is prevalent, are the lesions caused by rheumatic heart disease responsible for complications during pregnancy, when most of the cardiac alterations secondary to physiological changes in the different haemodynamic parameters manifest themselves. However, if patients do not recognise the abnormal symptoms and do not receive the appropriate study and treatment, their prognosis and the product of their pregnancy will be more reserved, despite the technology and human resources available.

The most common types of congenital heart disease in pregnancy are:

Atrial septal defect (ASD) If there is no pulmonary hypertension, pregnancy is well tolerated even if the defect is not corrected, although after the fourth decade the risk of supraventricular arrhythmias and the risk of paradoxical embolism increases.

Ventricular septal defect (VSD): If large and uncorrected, it can lead to heart failure (HF) and arrhythmias. If P.T.H. is present, the maternal risk is very high. If the I.V.C. is restrictive, pregnancy is usually well tolerated, although there is a risk of bacterial endocarditis. In cases of unrepaired I.V.C., postpartum severe hypotension due to bleeding and reversal of the shunt may occur, requiring volume and vasopressors for stabilisation.

Ductus: When it is small, there is only a risk of endocarditis. If it is large and has undergone surgery, it can be considered normal, although there may be sequelae of high pulmonary resistance or ventricular dilatation. When it is large and persistent, I.C. may appear and in this case rest and diuretics may be recommended, as well as assessing the need for closure. In the post-partum period, if P.T.H. is present, arterial hypotension may reverse the shunt, just as in I.V.C.

Aortic coarctation: Maternal complications are rare, but can be severe in those without A.T.H. surgery. Despite surgical correction in infancy and normalisation of the A.T., there is a risk of aortic dissection or rupture during pregnancy, especially in aortoplasties with Dacron patch, angioplasties with balloon catheter in native coarctation and associated with a bicuspid aorta. Other complications may include heart failure, A.T.H., angina and infective endocarditis. There is controversy as to whether termination of pregnancy should be by caesarean section or normal delivery.

Tetralogy of Fallot: This is the most experienced cyanotic CC in post-correction pregnancies. The risk is similar to the general population, especially if the residual lesions (pulmonary insufficiency and right ventricular outflow tract obstruction) are mild, if there is adequate ventricular function and there are no arrhythmias on exertion. Indicators of poor prognosis would be haematocrit > 60%, O2 saturation < 80%, right ventricular systolic pressure > 50% of systemic and history of syncope. Following this classification it can be stated that the two major groups of congenital heart disease in pregnancy are:

Repaired congenital heart disease: this is the ideal scenario, as every girl with CHD should undergo surgical and/or haemodynamic repair during childhood or adolescence, thus allowing the haemodynamic situation prior to surgical and/or haemodynamic repair to be restored.

The patient's haemodynamic status (often not compatible with life in complex CHD), restore normal haemodynamics and thus reach adulthood.

In particular, for women who have had their CC repaired, it allows them (depending on the CC) to carry a pregnancy into adulthood. However, this statement must be analysed with caution, as not all CHD are capable of carrying a normal pregnancy. In fact, after a CHD repair, there are often CHD residues, sequelae and complications that deteriorate the haemodynamic status of the woman. This is compounded by non-cardiovascular and acquired cardiovascular diseases, which add to morbidity.In summary, haemodynamic residues of CHD manifest as persistent shunts at different levels (atrial, ventricular, valvular) or extracardiac shunts that increase pulmonary flow, impair cardiac function, cause new valvular insufficiencies, and have a proarrhythmogenic effect, among other consequences.As previously described, during pregnancy, increased circulating volume, increased CO, would increase the haemodynamic effect of residual CHD (e.g. residual ventricular septal defect, residual valvular regurgitation, residual valvular stenosis), in general decreasing the ability of the cardiovascular system to adapt to the physiological changes that should normally be tolerated during pregnancy.

Unrepaired congenital heart disease: this scenario is not appropriate, as many women with CHD did not even know they had CHD. It is not uncommon for a CHD to be diagnosed for the first time in adult life, and just when it occurs in the setting of a CHD complication during the course of a pregnancy.

While many of the CHD first diagnosed in adulthood are simple or of medium complexity, it is not uncommon to find unrepaired complex CHD. Specifically in LATAM and Caribbean countries, the diagnosis of unrepaired CHD in adulthood can be as high as 30%. In short, all physiological haemodynamic changes will double or triple depending on the degree of haemodynamic impact of the unrepaired CHD. And depending on the type of CHD (cyanotic or non-cyanotic), some will not be able to continue gestation or will not be able to carry to term. This has consequences not only for the foetus, which in many cases ends up immature and dies, but also has serious consequences for maternal health.

Complex heart diseases

There is a group of more complex congenital heart diseases that are statistically rare, but which cause important clinical problems, such as tricuspid atresia, Ebstein's disease, single ventricle and truncus. In Presbitero 7's series of 96 pregnancies in44 patients with cyanotic CC, excluding the Eisenmenger situation, the frequency of maternal complications was 32%: heart failure, supraventricular paroxysmal tachycardia, thrombosis and endocarditis. The number of live newborns was 41 (43%), of which 15 (37%) were preterm.

Transposition of the great arteries: In patients operated with the Senning or Mustard technique, the main problem will be related to the tolerance of the V.D., which is subjected to systemic pressure, due to the volume overload caused by pregnancy. Ventricular atrial block may also be frequent. There is still little information on patients corrected with the Jatene technique (arterial switch).

Tricuspid atresia: With Fontan treatment, the woman can have a well-tolerated pregnancy, although the single ventricle must take on the volume overload. Complications may include C.I. or atrial flutter. In Canobio 10's series of 126 women operated with the Fontan technique, 38 pregnancies were recorded, with

45% live births, all of which were of low birth weight.

Ebstein's disease: Maternal complications will depend on the degree of tricuspid regurgitation, right ventricular dysfunction and cyanosis due to right-to-left atrial shunt. The more cyanosis, the greater the risk of paradoxical embolism, fetal hypoxaemia, endocarditis and right I.C. The incidence of paroxysmal supraventricular arrhythmias increases during pregnancy.

Eisenmenger's syndrome: As mentioned above, maternal mortality is significant and can reach 50%, as well as fetal risk of miscarriage, prematurity or low birth weight, so it is highly recommended to avoid pregnancy. Daliento studied the natural history and risk factors in 188 patients with Eisenmenger Syndrome, followed for 31 years and found a significant maternal mortality (27%) related to gestation, a high incidence of miscarriages (35.8%), as well as heart disease in the offspring (20%).

In case of pregnancy, early hospitalisation is recommended due to the risk of premature birth, and anticoagulant treatment during the last 8-10 weeks and 4 weeks postpartum.

Valvulopathies include the following listed:

Mitral Stenosis: The most frequent is of rheumatic origin. In mild or moderate Mitral Stenosis, treatment will be medical with diuretics to improve symptoms of pulmonary and venous congestion, and beta-blockers to decrease the maternal heart rate (H.F.) and thus prolong ventricular diastolic filling.

In cases of severe mitral stenosis (functional class III-IV and/or mitral area < 1cm2), mitral valvuloplasty (percutaneous or surgical) should be recommended prior to conception, as it considerably increases maternal and foetal risk. Vaginal delivery with haemodynamic monitoring should be advised, with maintenance up to several hours later, given the sudden increase in preload after delivery.

Mitral regurgitation: This will usually be caused by mitral valve prolapse and is usually well tolerated, given the reduction in systemic vascular resistance.

Medical management of symptomatic patients is based on diuretic treatment for pulmonary congestion and vasodilator treatment when accompanied by systemic AHT. It should be remembered that the
I.E.C.A.S. are contraindicated in pregnancy.

Aortic stenosis: The most common cause is congenital. It can worsen due to the physiological increase in preload and decrease in afterload that occurs in pregnancy, so when there is severe (gradient > 50 mmHg) or symptomatic stenosis, pregnancy should be avoided until it is corrected. Assessment of tolerance to pregnancy should be performed prior to conception by echocardiography and ergometry.

When stenosis is severe, even in asymptomatic women, there is a high risk during pregnancy of pulmonary oedema, angina, left I.C., sudden death and miscarriage. In cases of bicuspid valve there is an increased risk of aortic root dilatation, which would increase the likelihood of dissection in the third trimester of pregnancy.

Aortic insufficiency: When left ventricular function is preserved, it is usually well tolerated during pregnancy. It is usually due to a bicuspid valve or Marfan syndrome. Treatment, if necessary, will be with diuretics and vasodilators. I.E.C.A.S. should be avoided during pregnancy and replaced by nifedipine or hydralazine.

Marfan syndrome: Women with this entity often have progressive aortic dilatation with aortic insufficiency, and mitral prolapse leading to mitral insufficiency (M.I.). The most important complications are aortic dissection and aortic rupture. If pregnancy is a possibility, the aortic root should be assessed, as a diameter > 4-5 cm is associated with a higher risk of fatal complications, and pregnancy would therefore be discouraged. During pregnancy, serial echocardiograms are recommended even if aortic size is normal, physical activity is restricted and beta-blocker treatment is recommended, if necessary, to prevent progressive aortic dilatation. At the time of delivery, general anaesthesia and caesarean section seem advisable to avoid sudden increases in blood pressure.

Valve prostheses

Maternal mortality is estimated at 1-4% in mechanical prosthesis wearers and is related to valve thrombosis. Hypercoagulable state increases the risk of thromboembolism. There will be an added foetal risk from anticoagulants.

The use of anticoagulants in pregnant women with prostheses is essential due to the increased risk of thromboembolism. However, the type of anticoagulation is controversial, there are different guidelines and a consensus must be reached with the pregnant woman on the type of guideline to follow.

Dicoumarinic drugs are the ones that best protect women against the risk of thrombosis, but during the first 6-10 weeks of pregnancy they can cause embryopathy in the foetus. Also at the end of gestation they have a risk of foetal loss or massive bleeding in the woman during delivery. Heparin s.c. or i.v. is indicated to avoid the risk of embryopathy but in the pregnant woman it can cause thrombocytopenia, osteoporosis, haematomas or sterile abscesses. Low molecular weight heparin does not affect the foetus but like sodium heparin it has a risk of thrombopenia and there is no literature to demonstrate its usefulness in pregnant women with mechanical prostheses, although it is widely used in autoimmune pathology.

However, there is a group of cardiac lesions that cannot be detected prenatally:

- Patent ductus arteriosus.
- Atrial septal defect of the ostium secundum type.
- Mild/moderate obstructions of the great vessels (aortic stenosis, pulmonary stenosis and coarctation of the aorta).
- Some ventricular septal defects.

Frequent maternal indications for fetal echocardiography and approximate risk of fetal heart defect (Mendoza-Calderón, et. al., (2012) & Mayorga, et. al., 2013).

1) Family history

a. One previous child affected (~2%)

b. Two children affected (~10%)

c. Maternal heart disease (~4%)

d. Paternal heart disease (~2%)

e. Genetic syndromes (variable)

2) Pre-existing maternal metabolic disease

a. Diabetes Mellitus (4-6%)

b. Phenylketonuria (12-16%)

3) Maternal infections

a. Parvovirus B19

b. Rubella

c. Coxsackie

4) Exposure to teratogens

a. Retinoids

b. Phenytoin

c. Carbamazepine

d. Valproic acid

e. Lithium

f.Alcohol

5) Maternal antibodies

a. Anti-Ro (SSA) and Anti-La (SSB)

Contraception in women with heart disease

It is an essential tool to prevent unplanned pregnancies or to make termination of pregnancy mandatory. No contraceptive is ideal for a woman with heart disease and the following aspects should be taken into account:

▪ Natural" and barrier methods are not recommended because of their high failure rate.

▪ Combined oral contraceptives are contraindicated if there is a risk of thromboembolism, due to the thrombotic risk of oestrogens.

▪ Contraceptives with progestogens alone do not increase the risk of thrombosis and have few side effects (irregular metrorrhagia), but their efficacy is lower than that of combined contraceptives. The use of intramuscular progestogens may be considered, especially in adolescents who are unsure whether they will maintain daily treatment with oral medication.

▪ Progestogen-releasing intrauterine devices are an important advance, as they are highly effective, do not increase the risk of thrombosis and reduce menstrual bleeding.

▪ Definitive sterilisation methods should be considered for women at high risk of pregnancy or when the couple has completed their desire to have children (Román Rubio, et. al., (2010) & 25. Fayad Saeta, et. al., (2009).

Cardiovascular risk stratification and grading

Ideally, every woman of childbearing age who is a carrier and survivor of a CHD repair should have a pre-gestational risk in her medical history that has been duly pre-established by her treating cardiologist at ACC. This pre-gestational risk is determined based on the type of CHD, current clinical status, NYHA (New York Heart Association) functional class, among other variables. Different scales and scores are available to calculate and establish the risk of adverse complications during pregnancy and CHD. Among them is the

CARPREG I and II (Cardiac disease in pregnancy) risk score, which determines four predictors of maternal complications: previous cardiac events, NYHA functional class > II or cyanosis, left heart obstruction and myocardial dysfunction. Adverse cardiac events are 5, 27 and 75% when, respectively, no factor is present, one factor is present and more than one risk factor is present.

The ZAHARA risk score [(Zwangerschap bij aangeboren hartafwijking) (Pregnancy in women with congenital heart disease)], also allows the frequency of adverse cardiac events to be calculated17. But the most comprehensive and widely used is the modified World Health Organization (mWHO) gestational risk classification scale, which seems to be more objective and easier to apply.

In addition to the mWHO scale, we recommend from the ACC chapter and the Pediatric Cardiology Council of the Interamerican Society of Cardiology (SIAC) to know and apply the criteria of the Anatomic and Physiological Classification in Adults with Congenital Heart Disease [(CAF-ACC) (APC-ACHD)], which was proposed in the 2018 American Heart Association and American College of Cardiology (AHA/ACC) guidelines in Adult Congenital Heart Disease 2018.

The CAF-ACC integrates the anatomy or morphology of the repaired or unrepaired CHD with the NYHA (New York Heart Association) functional class and the combination with 9 clinical variables, which, if present or not, add morbidity. These clinical variables are: hypoxaemia, pulmonary arterial hypertension, haemodynamically significant defect, venous and arterial stenosis, capacity, and the presence or absence of a pulmonary arterial hypertension. exercise, target organ dysfunction, concomitant acquired valvular disease, arrhythmia and aortopathy.

The combination of the type of CHD (simple, medium or high complexity) whether repaired or not repaired added to the NYHA functional class (I, II, III and IV) and the variables present in the woman with CHD finally determines 4 CAF-ACC states, which in their respective order of lesser to greater severity are: A, B, C and D.The ACC chapter and the Paediatric Cardiology Council of the SIAC recommend, in addition to applying the mWHO scale, to combine it with the application of the CAF-ACC, thus obtaining the highest degree of objective accuracy in classifying gestational risk in women with CHD. By establishing CAF-ACC and mWHO risk, changes in gestational evolution can be determined, allowing us to determine clinical behaviour and thus establish a plan for delivery care and haemodynamic monitoring. This more precise objectivity of risk stratification also allows us to anticipate and avoid serious haemodynamic consequences in the immediate postpartum and early puerperium, where most complications occur in women with CHD. This ensures adequate maternal and infant care.

Special considerations

All pregnancies with pulmonary hypertension (PH) should be closely monitored with advanced therapies, and delivery should be with a multidisciplinary team experienced in PH20. As a general rule, pregnancy is absolutely contraindicated in the presence of Eisenmenger's syndrome. In case of severe cyanosis (SO2 < 85%) pregnancy is not recommended.

In case of mechanical valves, vitamin K antagonists should be switched to some form of low molecular weight heparin during the first trimester. Then, during the second trimester, vitamin K antagonists can be switched back to vitamin K antagonists up to 36 weeks, to avoid thrombosis from heparin.

Studies assessing the usefulness of adverse pregnancy outcomes in vascular disease risk stratification

Relatively few published studies have rigorously evaluated the utility of adding a history of adverse pregnancy outcomes to conventional vascular disease risk stratification. These studies suggest that, although adverse pregnancy outcomes may be a factor for early development of vascular disease, they may not contribute substantially to the prediction of VE or to the net reclassification of VE when taking into account established RV factors.

In fact, it may be that the burden of adverse pregnancy outcomes as a vascular risk factor may be confounded by the Diabetes Mellitus, hypertension and dyslipidaemia already present. Previous studies have evaluated the additional information provided by the following adverse pregnancy outcomes: fetal loss, hypertensive disorders of pregnancy, preterm delivery and pre-eclampsia, pre-eclampsia, gestational hypertension, preterm delivery or delivery of small-for-gestational-age fetus. The predictive ability that adverse pregnancy outcomes may add may be limited by their lower prevalence compared to traditional vascular risk factors and the more current data provided by classical vascular risk factors. In addition, studies of vascular event risk stratification by considering adverse pregnancy outcomes have been conducted in middle-aged and older women, stages where it is more likely that conventional vascular risk factors may have already developed, limiting the potential contribution of adverse pregnancy outcomes in identifying women at higher long-term risk of vascular events.

Lifestyle modification for the reduction of rae in women with pregnancy-related disorders as a first measure

It is essential to establish health promotion policies and healthy environments that promote healthy lifestyles, modifying risk factors such as physical inactivity, unhealthy diet, tobacco and alcohol consumption, exposure to air and noise pollution (especially from road traffic), and acting on climate change.

In other words, making healthy easy, creating environments where the default options are health-promoting. Recommendations for promoting physical activity and reducing sedentary lifestyles include urban planning measures that facilitate active and healthy mobility, active transport and increasing the availability of spaces and facilities that facilitate physical activity in schools and community settings.Promoting healthy eating includes legislative measures to ban or reduce trans fats, reduce calorie intake, salt, added sugars and saturated fats in prepared foods and beverages, fiscal measures (taxation or incentives) on some foods and beverages, and the availability of healthy meals in the menus served and in food vending machines in the school and work environment. It also includes recommendations, mainly legislative, to reduce tobacco and alcohol consumption: regulation of consumption in public places; availability and sale; advertising; labelling and packaging; pricing policies and the implementation of educational campaigns. Finally, measures are recommended to reduce emissions of small particulate and gaseous pollutants, the use of solid fuels and road traffic, as well as limiting carbon dioxide emissions to reduce morbidity and mortality from vascular events. The population-based approach can bring numerous benefits, such as reducing the gap in health inequalities, preventing other non-communicable diseases that have common risk factors and determinants with vascular events, such as cancer, lung disease and type 2 diabetes mellitus, as well as saving the health and social costs of avoided vascular events.

It is also necessary to understand that living conditions and the social determinants of health not only determine different vascular risk, but also different access to prevention and promotion measures. It is therefore key to maintain an equity approach (including a gender approach) in the development of strategies or interventions.Dietary patterns to optimise vascular health in women of reproductive age, and pregnant women. Healthy dietary patterns can optimise vascular health for all women, which may be especially important before pregnancy. Epidemiological cohort studies suggest that healthy dietary patterns up to three years before pregnancy (i.e. characterised by a high intake of fruits, vegetables and legumes, nuts and fish, and a low intake of red and processed meats) are associated with a lower risk of hypertensive disorders of pregnancy, gestational diabetes and preterm birth. Maternal nutrition in the twelve months prior to conception can affect fetal growth and development, as well as gestational age and birth weight. Among women with uncomplicated pregnancies, the DASH (Dietary Approaches to Stop Hypertension) diet was associated with lower blood pressure than other dietary patterns.A diet rich in protein and fruit was associated with a lower risk of preterm birth, while a diet high in fat and sugar was associated with a higher risk of preterm birth. Among women with gestational diabetes, the DASH diet was associated with better pregnancy outcomes, including lower insulin requirements. Following the DASH diet during pregnancy was associated with a lower risk of preterm birth according to a cohort study. Although these associations could be confounded by other favourable medical and lifestyle factors, it seems clear that recommending the consumption of a healthy diet, such as the Mediterranean diet, is an appropriate health programme.Special considerations for optimising dietary intake in women of reproductive age and pregnant women with gestational diabetes or pre-eclampsia. It is recommended that women of reproductive age consume folic acid and iron supplements in addition to a healthy dietary pattern.

Prophylaxis of iron deficiency anaemia during pregnancy is based on ensuring 30 mg of elemental iron per day during pregnancy in singleton pregnancies and 60 mg/day in multiple pregnancies.

During lactation the intake should be 15 mg/day during breastfeeding. A balanced diet of iron-rich foods (beef, chicken, turkey or pork, fish, vegetables [spinach and chard], legumes [lentils], nuts and fortified cereals) is recommended, along with oral iron supplementation at low doses from the 20th week of gestation in women who are found to have inadequate iron stores.

In pregnant women at risk of iron deficiency anaemia such as multiple pregnancies, gastrointestinal surgery, iron-poor diets, adolescents or those with short inter-gestational periods of less than one year, a specific study by means of a ferric profile can be assessed and supplementation can be considered if iron deficiency anaemia is confirmed. Supplements should preferably be taken at bedtime or between meals together with vitamin C to favour their absorption, as long as side effects permit, and should not be taken with tea, milk or coffee. Some commentary suggests that universal iron supplementation for healthy women with adequate nutrition and normal iron status is not necessary and may not be safe, advising that supplementation should be tailored to individual needs.

In Spain, the General Directorate of Public Health of the then Ministry of Health and Consumer Affairs advises that women without a history of a pregnancy affected by a Neural Tube Defect (NTD) who are planning a pregnancy should take 0.4 mg/day of folic acid, while those with a history of a pregnancy affected by NTD should take 4 mg/day of folic acid, in both cases from at least one month before pregnancy and during the first three months of pregnancy, in addition to a diet with foods rich in folic acid (NE=Ia-A).

Adherence to dietary and physical activity recommendations may reduce the risk of developing gestational diabetes. Increased risk of developing type 2 diabetes among women who had gestational diabetes suggests that the adoption of a healthy diet may be particularly valuable in preventing late-onset diabetes.

Although a high level of evidence documents the beneficial effect of a healthy dietary pattern in lowering blood pressure in the general population, there are inconsistent data on its value in preventing the development of chronic hypertension after pre-eclampsia. Future clinical trials could investigate the efficacy of dietary changes in preventing the development of risk factors for CVD in women who have experienced an RAE, particularly gestational diabetes and hypertensive disorders of pregnancy.

Physical activity to optimise vascular health in women of reproductive age and pregnant women. Maternal obesity and excessive gestational weight gain are associated in the short term with difficulties in breastfeeding (which, as reviewed in this paper, has protective effects on cardio-metabolic health) and, in the long term, with postpartum weight retention, type 2 diabetes and increased risks of subsequent hypertensive disorders of pregnancy. Preconception obesity and excessive gestational weight gain also lead to increased risks of adverse adiposity-related outcomes for offspring, such as higher childhood BMI and total and abdominal body fat mass, cardio-metabolic risks such as childhood hypertension, changes in cardiac structure and altered biochemical parameters such as high insulin and triglyceride levels, as well as low HDL-cholesterol levels.

Interventions led by health professionals may have greater efficacy in weight reduction than those led by non-health professionals, and diet and supervised exercise combined showed greater average weight reduction in a meta-analysis concluding that diet and/or physical activity-based interventions during pregnancy reduce excessive gestational weight gain and also reduce the likelihood of caesarean section, with no evidence that the effects differed between subgroups of women.

However, to achieve a greater population impact, intersectoral and interdisciplinary work at community and local level is key. In uncomplicated pregnancies, the recommendation would be moderate-intensity physical activity for at least 150 minutes of moderate physical activity distributed throughout the week, according to the recommendations of the World Health Organisation and the Ministry of Health.

Women who are sedentary before pregnancy should gradually increase their physical activity. Similarly, 150 min/week of moderate-intensity aerobic activity is recommended during pregnancy and postpartum, followed by a gradual increase in physical activity. vigorous physical activity in women who were already active before pregnancy. It is not recommended to start vigorous-intensity physical activity during pregnancy if the woman was previously inactive. Moderate-intensity physical activity during lactation does not affect the quantity or composition of milk or the growth of the infant. Other lifestyle factors. Any use of intoxicants (tobacco, alcohol, other drugs) during gestation and postpartum is strongly discouraged due to their adverse short- and long-term effects on fetal health, including preterm delivery, fetal growth restriction/low birth weight, sudden infant death syndrome, neurodevelopmental and behavioural problems, fetal alcohol spectrum disorders, obesity, hypertension, type 2 diabetes, impaired lung function or asthma. These recommendations also influence the reduction of VE in women with smoking-related EAR, as smoking is one of the most important modifiable risk factors in premenopausal women.

The area of sleep and postpartum stress, including depression, anxiety and subsequent vascular disease in women, has not been well studied, but represents an important area for future research and a potential opportunity for future lifestyle recommendations unique to women of childbearing age.

METHOD

A case series study was conducted during the period January to December 2015 in the Cardiopathy and Pregnancy Department of the General University Hospital "Vladimir Ilich Lenin", Holguín Province, with the aim of contributing to the Maternal and Infant programme to a better understanding of the evolution of pregnancy in patients with heart disease. The study universe consisted of pregnant women with heart disease who were seen at the Cardiopathy and Pregnancy Clinic during the study period. Pregnant women with heart disease were considered to be those with a previous diagnosis, confirmed diagnosis or first diagnosis of a cardiac lesion, according to the anamnesis and complementary examinations. The diagnosis and clinical follow-up was carried out by two cardiologists from the hospital's cardiology service with the support of an obstetrician-gynecologist in defining the final course of action.As complementary examinations, each patient underwent a 12-lead surface E.K.G. with Cardiocid BB A5102 equipment and an M, 2D and Doppler echocardiogram with Prosound Alfa10 Premier equipment. Follow-up was performed according to the New York Heart Association functional classification: monthly for classes III and IV and quarterly for classes I and II. The variables considered were recorded. When necessary, complementary tests were repeated.

The New York Heart Association criteria were used to determine the functional capacity of the patients:

- Grade I: No limitations to physical activity.
- Grade II: mild limitation of physical activity.
- Grade III: marked limitation of physical activity. Recovers during rest.
- Grade IV: Incapacity for physical activity at the slightest exertion, heart failure is present.

Cases were excluded from the study if they did not meet the diagnostic criteria for heart disease and/or had dropped out of follow-up at their own request or had been transferred to another province.

To achieve the first specific objective, variables were defined according to the type of specific cardiac lesion: congenital, rheumatic and others; with information from the clinical histories of each patient. For the determination of the time of diagnosis of heart disease, we defined whether the diagnosis was made before or during pregnancy; we also considered the time at which the obstetric advice given by the attending physician and the advice given by the cardiologist regarding pregnancy or continuation of pregnancy, termination of pregnancy or prohibition of pregnancy was reported. A cardiac complication was considered to be a cardiac complication if at any time during pregnancy or puerperium: cardiac dysrhythmias, acute pulmonary oedema, infective endocarditis or other requiring medical intervention and treatment. Information was collected from the patients' medical records.

The period of pregnancy was considered in first, second and third trimester, during labour and puerperium, which allowed for adequate interpretation and comparison of the information with other studies. The final route of delivery was defined as euthecological, instrumental or caesarean delivery, specifying in the case of dystocia whether the cause was obstetric or cardiac.

Perinatal morbimortality was considered; birth weight less than 2500 grams, severe hypoxia, foetal deaths or deceased newborns; all these variables related to the mother's pathology. The information will be taken from the obstetric medical records at delivery. Collected by means of a questionnaire, drawn up by the author and tutor, which provided an output for the objectives set, the information being completed with a review of the clinical histories. An automated database was created with the information; the database was interrogated according to the output tables drawn up in response to the objectives. To carry out the study, the Windows Vista Ultímate operating system was used on a P5 PC. The calculations of the different parameters and statistical tests, as well as their analysis, were carried out using the statistical package of the Excel software or Microsoft Office tabulator.

The results were presented in contingency tables of columns and rows, using absolute frequencies to describe the pregnant women with congenital or acquired heart disease according to the variables studied, and the percentage was used as a summary measure of qualitative variables and was organised on a nominal and ordinal scale, which were computer-processed. Statistics such as mean and standard deviation were used for the variable age. The results were analysed using the statistical programme MedCalc®.

Main variables:

- Category.
- Heart Injury.
- Diagnosis.
- Orientation.

- Functional Capacity.
- Complications.
- Momentum.
- The birth canal.
- Morbidity and mortality.

Operationalisation of Variables and Definition of Scales.

Variable	Type of Variable	Operationalisation	
		Scale	Description
Diagnostic Category	Qualitative Nominal	Rheumatic	nflammatory, non-suppurative ecurrent inflammatory disease caused by the immune itis caused by group A beta olytic streptococcus, which from two to three months of age, is a or three weeks of causing acute pharyngotonsillitis, the main organ affected being the heart.
		Congenital	-When the disease is due to a problem of foetal development and maturation
		Other	- Any other cause
		Rheumatic:	-When taking into account that the relevant entity is of rheumatic cause
		Mitral Stenosis	
		Mitral Insufficiency	
		Mitral Disease	
		Mitroaortic disease	
		Aortic insufficiency	
		Aortic Stenosis	
Heart Injury	Qualitative Nominal	Congenital: Aorta Bicuspid Aorta CIV	-When it is taken into account that the corresponding entity is congenital in cause
		CIA	
		Pulmonary Stenosis	
		Others:	
		Valve Prolapse	
		Mitral	
		Heart surgery	
		Pre-excitation	
		Peripartum cardiomyopathy	--When it is taken into account that the corresponding entity is of any other non-rheumatic or non-congenital cause

Diagnosis of Heart Disease	Qualitative Nominal	Before Pregnancy During Pregnancy	-Previous period when the woman is not pregnant -Period at on that the woman at is in the making
Orientation	Qualitative Nominal	You canget pregnantor continue pregnancy Cannot impregnate Terminate the pregnancy Did not receive the advice	-If the patient is able to become pregnant or continue the pregnancy -If the patient is unable to become pregnant -If the pregnancy has to be terminated -If the patient did not receive counselling
		Grade I	-No physical limitation of movement, no symptoms with routine physical activity, despite ventricular dysfunction (confirmed e.g. by echocardiography). -Symptoms appear with ordinary daily physical activity (e.g. climbing stairs) resulting in fatigue, dyspnoea, palpitations. They disappear with rest or minimal physical activity, when the patient becomes more comfortable. -There is marked exercise limitation. Symptoms appear with minor physical activities (such as walking). They disappear with rest. -Inability to perform any physical activity. Appears symptoms even at rest.
		Grade II	
Functional Capacity	Qualitative Ordinal		
		Grade III	
		Grade IV	
Complications	Qualitative Nominal	Cardiac arrhythmias	-Heart rhythm disorders, it is a alteration of the heart rate, either because it speeds up, slows down or slows down.
		Acute Lung Oedema Infective Endocarditis	irregular heartbeat, which occurs when there are abnormalities in the electrical conduction system of the heart. -Fluid accumulation in the lungs with interstitial oedema and lymphatic insufficiency of cardiac origin -Inflammatory process located in the inner lining of native or prosthetic chambers and valves. cardiac

Timing of Presentation of Complications	Qualitative Ordinal	First Trimester Second Trimester Third Trimester During Childbirth During the Puerperium	-The first three months of pregnancy -The second three months of pregnancy -The third three months of pregnancy -Time in which the birth takes place -Time after delivery
Childbirth Pathway	Qualitative Nominal	Euthyroid Instrumented Caesarean Section	-Normal delivery -Surgical delivery -Birth with need instrumentation
Morbidity and mortality	Qualitative Nominal	Prematurity Severe Hypoxia at Birth	Birth before 36.6 weeks gestation Decrease of oxygen values below normal limits

Ethical aspects

- World Medical Association criteria (Helsinki Protocol) in its current version for research in humans, based on the principles of autonomy, beneficence, justice and non-maleficence as a way of guaranteeing the ethical protection of the patients under study.

- The possibility of withdrawing from the study at any time without affecting the quality of medical care required by patients.

ANALYSIS AND DISCUSSION OF THE RESULTS

The increase in the number of pregnant women with heart disease who are evaluated at the heart disease and pregnancy clinic of the ¨Vladimir Ilich Lenin¨ General University Hospital with a rigorous cardiological and obstetric assessment has led to a rapid diagnosis of heart disease, which in the non-pregnant state goes unnoticed.

Table 1. Distribution of cases according to diagnostic category of origin.

Category	№	%
Other	23	38,3
Congenital	19	31,7
Rheumatic	18	30
Total	60	100

Source: Database.

When analysing the main heart diseases associated with pregnancy according to diagnostic category (Table 1), the highest number of cases was observed in the other category with 23 (38.3%).In the results, congenital and rheumatic lesions are practically equal because the natural rate of the latter decreases while that of the former remains relatively constant (0.8*100 live births), due to the improvement of congenital cardiopathies that allows a larger population of patients with heart disease to reach reproductive age and to the decrease in the incidence of rheumatic fever due to greater prophylactic and therapeutic control (González Maqueda, et. al., 2000).The results of the research are in line with the literature reviewed, which suggests a predominance of congenital heart disease. According to the literature consulted and authors such as Manso, et. al. (2008), Thorne, et. al. (2006), & Regitz-Zagrosek, et. al. (2014), currently in developed countries, the main cause of cardiovascular disease in pregnancy is congenital in origin, due to the near disappearance of rheumatic fever and the improvement in the care and surgical management of these patients. Other causes, although less frequent, include hypertensive, ischaemic, syphilitic and cardiomyopathies, among others.

Table 2. Distribution of cases according to specific cardiac lesion

Lesión cardiaca	№	%
*Congénitas		
-Aorta Bicúspide	2	3,30
-CIV	9	15,0
-CIA	5	8,30
-Estenosis Pulmonar	3	5,00
*Reumáticas		
-Estenosis Mitral	8	13,3
-Insuficiencia Mitral	5	8,30
-Enfermedad Mitral	2	3,30
-Enfermedad Mitroaortica	1	1,70
-Insuficiencia Aortica	1	1,70
-Estenosis Aortica	1	1,70
*Otras		
-Prolapso de la Válvula Mitral	13	21,7
-Operadas del Corazón	6	10,0
-Pre Excitación	2	3,30
- Miocardiopatía periparto	2	3,30
Total	**60**	**100.0**

Source: Database.

Table 2 shows the cases according to specific cardiac lesion. Here it can be seen that the most frequent heart diseases were; mitral valve prolapse 13 patients (21.7%), mitral stenosis 8 patients (13.3%) and mitral insufficiency 5 cases (8.3%). The results coincide with those reported by other authors such as Mendoza-Calderón, et. al., (2012), Botella Llusiá (1984), & Aguilera Castro, et. al., (2012); who point out the predominance of pregnant women with mitral valve involvement.It cannot be overemphasised that the most frequent cardiac lesion identified in the study was mitral valve prolapse, which is related to the development of echocardiography and the high scientific level reached by health professionals. It should be noted that 10% of the pregnant women (6 cases) had undergone previous heart surgery, and in none of the cases were there any complications. Regarding the results of the casuistry studied, in the aforementioned bibliography there are contradictions between different authors who state that mitral valve prolapse occupies first place with a prevalence of 0.5 to 5 % in the general population, between 6 -10 % in young women, and 21 % in women of reproductive age, which could explain the results, in addition, 6 % of echocardiograms in young women, supposedly normal, give a diagnosis of mitral valve prolapse; These estimates place it among the most frequent clinical heart disease, and some studies have even identified it as the most frequent valvular heart disease.

Table 3. Time of diagnosis of heart disease

Diagnosis	№	%
Before Pregnancy	51	85
During Pregnancy	9	15
Total	60	100
Source: Database.		

When analysing the time of diagnosis of heart disease (Table 3), 51 cases (85%) were diagnosed before pregnancy and only 15% (9 cases) were diagnosed during pregnancy. In the literature reviewed, authors such as Valladares-Carvajal, et. al., (2011) & Mendoza-Calderón, et. al., (2012) report a low percentage of diagnosis during pregnancy. Primary care physicians play an important role in the early diagnosis and appropriate treatment of pregnant women with heart disease. Therefore, the results could be related to better preconception risk management, which allows for the diagnosis of any pre-pregnancy heart disease.

Table 4. Counselling offered in obstetric counselling.

Orientación	Médico de asistencia		Especialista cardiología	
	№	%	№	%
Puede embarazar o Continuar embarazo	9	15	56	93,3
No puede embarazar	47	78,3	1	1,7
Interrumpir el embarazo	4	6,7	3	5
No recibió consejo	---	---	---	---
Total	**60**	**100**	**60**	**100**

Source: Survey.

Table 4 shows the guidance offered in obstetric counselling to pregnant women by the attending physician and the cardiology specialist. Unacceptably, 78.3% of pregnant women with heart disease (47 cases) reported that their attending physician advised them that they could not become pregnant and only 9 cases (15%) could become pregnant. However, in cardiology consultations 93.3% of the pregnant women (56 cases) were advised that they could become pregnant or continue the pregnancy and only 5% of the cases were advised to terminate the pregnancy because they had severe valvular heart disease with risk to their lives.

In the literature reviewed, no studies were found that addressed this discrepancy in terms of obstetric advice between the attending physician and the cardiology specialist, which could be related to the primary health care approach to the control of perinatal morbidity and mortality.It is important to reaffirm that termination of pregnancy carries risks and if there is no contraindication and the appropriate conditions exist, it is preferable not to indicate termination.

Table 5. Classification of patients according to the functional capacity of their heart disease.

Functional capacity	№	%
I	48	80,0
II	8	13,3
III	3	5
IV	1	1,70
Total	60	100
Source: Database.		
In establishing the classification of	cardiac patients according to	functional capacity (Table 5) is

This predominance could be related to the higher frequency of these groups in heart disease in general; and taking into account that functional capacity III and IV present a higher risk of maternal and foetal mortality, pregnancy is more frequently avoided in these patients. The results agree with Drenthen, et. al., (2005), Rendón, (2014) where a predominance of grade I is also shown.

Table 6. Cardiac complications in pregnant women.

Complications	№	%
Cardiac dysrhythmias	2	66,7
Acute lung oedema	1	33,3
Infective endocarditis	---	---
Total	3	100

Source: Database.

Cardiovascular complications encountered (Table 6) included arrhythmias, 2 cases with paroxysmal supraventricular tachycardia, which accounted for 66.7% of complications, and one case with acute pulmonary oedema (33.3%). In the literature reviewed, Alonso Gómez, et. al., (2012) & Pijuan Domènecha, et. al., (2006), report higher figures for complications. Other authors report an incidence of complications similar to ours. The haemodynamic overload caused by pregnancy together with the compromise implied by vascular damage could explain the incidence of electrical and haemodynamic complications that should be taken into account in the follow-up of pregnant women with heart disease. Adequate follow-up of cardiac patients before, during and after delivery by a multidisciplinary team resulted in a low rate of complications.

Table 7. Relationship between functional capacity and cardiovascular complications.

Functional capacity №		Complications №	%
I	48	---	---
II	8	---	---
III	3	2	66,7
IV	1	1	100
Total	60	3	5

Source: Database.

When establishing the relationship between functional capacity and the occurrence of complications (Table 7), it can be seen that the highest percentage of complications occurred in functional capacities IV (100%) and III (66.7%). This shows that the greater the deterioration in functional physical capacity, the greater the risk of pregnancy complications. The results were similar to those of other authors, who also report a higher percentage of complications in patients with functional capacity III and IV.

Table 8. Timing of complications

Moment	Complications	
	№	%
First trimester	----	----
Second quarter	----	----
Third trimester	2	66,7
During childbirth	----	----
During the postpartum period	1	33,3
Total	3	100

Source: Database.

An analysis of the timing of complications (Table 8) shows that the highest percentage of 2 cases (66.7%) occurred in the third trimester and 1 case (33.3%) in the puerperium.Cardiovascular complications can appear in any trimester of pregnancy, but in the third trimester the haemodynamic load is greater, which means that they appear more frequently during this stage. The paper agrees with several authors Drenthen, et. al., (2005), Conte, et. al., (2002) and others such as Thaman, et. al., (2009), Melvin, et. al., (2009), report the highest percentage of complications during the first trimester of pregnancy.

Table 9. Final route of delivery in pregnant women according to obstetric or cardiac cause

Category Obstetric cause Cardiac cause

№		%	№	%	№		%
Euthyphilic	39	65	---	---	---		---
Caesarean section	12	20	12	100	---		---
Instrumented	9	15	7	77,8		3	33,3
Total	60	100	19	31,7		3	5,0

Source: Database.

Table 9 shows the final route of delivery in pregnant women. Euthocic delivery predominated in 39 cases, 5%. 100% of the caesarean deliveries (12 cases) were due to obstetric causes and 77.8% of the instrumented deliveries were also due to obstetric causes. Three deliveries 33.3% of the instrumented deliveries were performed at the indication of the cardiologist with the aim of shortening labour time.In the literature reviewed, there is a coincidence of criteria in that delivery should preferably be vaginal, with as short a labour time as possible; and instrumentation should only be indicated in cases that require it, and caesarean section should only be performed if possible for obstetric or cardiological reasons (Manso, et. al., 2008). The results were similar to those reported by Schlemmer, (1995) & Acho-Mego, (2011), regarding the predominance of euthyphal delivery.

Table 10. Indicators of perinatal morbidity and mortality in the studied cases

Morbidity and mortality	№	%*
Prematurity	2	3,3
Severe hypoxia at birth	2	3,3
Total	4	6,6

Source: Database.*---% in relation to the total number of pregnant women.

When analysing the perinatal morbidity and mortality of the cases studied (Table 10), 2 preterm births were found (3.3%). No cases of perinatal and maternal mortality were reported. The medical literature highlights the negative influence of heart disease on the product of conception as an indicator of low birth weight. The results indicate very low rates of prematurity and no maternal or neonatal deaths (Fayad Saeta, et. al., (2009) & Emergency Cardiac Care Committee (2009).

CONCLUSIONS

To raise the level of medical knowledge in primary health care about the pathophysiology of cardiac disorders during pregnancy by means of advanced training courses, which will make it possible to establish an adequate selection of patients who may or may not conceive their pregnancy and at the same time increase the screening for heart disease in the prenatal stage.

BIBLIOGRAPHICAL REFERENCES

1. Manso B, Pijuán A, Giralt G, Ferrer Q, Betrián P, et al. Pregnancy and congenital heart disease. Rev Esp Cardiol [Internet]. 2008 [Cited 12 Nov 2015]; 61(3): [Approx 8 p.]. Available at: http://www.revespcardiol.org/es/embarazo-cardiopatias-congenitas/articulo/13116650/

2. Thorne S, MacGregor A, Nelson-Piercy C. Risk of contraception and pregnancy in heart disease. Heart [Internet]. 2006 [Cited Nov 12, 2015]; 92(5): [Approx 6 p.]. Available from: http://www.ncbi.nlm.nih.gov/pmc/articles/PMC1861048/

3. Drenthen W, Pieper P, Ploeg M, Voors A, Roos-Hesselink J, Mulder B, et al. Risk of complication during pregnancy after Senning or Mustard repair of complete transposition of the great arteries. Eur Heart J [Internet]. 2005 [Cited Sept 4, 2015]; 26(13): [Approx 8 p.]. Available from: http://eurheartj.oxfordjournals.org/content/26/23/2588.long.

4. Rendón Iván D, Soto M, Jaramillo M, Palacio AC, Restrepo JA. Tetralogy of Fallot and pregnancy. Rev Colomb Cardiol [Internet]. 2014 Aug [cited 2016 Sep 22]; 21(4): [Approx 5 p.]. Available from: http://dx.doi.org/10.1016/j.rccar.2014.04.002.

5. Regitz-Zagrosek V, Blomstrom Lundqvist C, Borghi C, Cifkova R, Ferreira R, Foidart JM. ESC clinical practice guideline for the management of cardiovascular disease during pregnancy. Rev Esp Cardiol [Internet]. 2014 [Cited Nov 10, 2015]; 65(2): [Approx 7 p.]. Available from: http://www.revespcardiol.org/es/guia-practica-clinica-esc- el/article/90093017/.

6. Bouzas B, Gatzoulis MA. Pulmonary arterial hypertension in adults with congenital heart disease. Rev Esp Cardiol [Internet]. 2005 [Cited 12 Nov 2015]; 58(11): [Approx 5p.].465-469. Available at: http://www.revespcardiol.org/es/hipertension-arterial-pulmonar-adultos-con/article/13074838/.

7. Román Rubio PA, Pérez Torga JE, Guerra Chang E, Couret Cabrera MP, Nodarse A, Sanabria AM. Eisenmenger's syndrome and pregnancy. Rev Cubana Obstet Ginecol [Internet]. 2011 Aug [cited2016 Sep22];37(2): [Approx 8 p.]. Available from: http://scielo.sld.cu/scielo.php?script=sci_arttext&pid=S0138-600X2011000200013&lng=es.

8. Mendoza-Calderón S A, Hernández-Pacheco J A, Estrada-Altamirano A, Nares-Torices MÁ, Orozco Méndez H, Hernández-Muñoz VA. Initial

evaluation of congenital heart disease with short circuit in pregnancy. Perinatol. Reprod. [Internet]. 2012 Sep [cited 2016Sep22]; 26(3):[Approx 12 p.].Available from: http://www.scielo.org.mx/scielo.php?script=sci_arttext&pid=S0187-53372012000300007&lng=es.

9. Botella Llusiá J, Clavero Núñez JA. Diseases that complicate gestation. In: Tratado de Ginecologia. Havana: Científico Técnica; 1984. p. 111-28.

10. Chio Naranjo I, Guerra Chang E, Yanes Calderón M, Román Rubio P, Pérez Torga JE, Pérez Felpeto R. Impact of pregnancy in pregnant women diagnosed with congenital heart disease. Rev Cubana Obstet Ginecol [Internet]. 2012 Jun [cited 2016 Sep 22] ; 38(2): [Approx 12 p.]. Available from: http://scielo.sld.cu/scielo.php?script=sci_arttext&pid=S0138-600X2012000200004&lng=en.

11. Conte MR, Piccininno M· Bernabò P· Bonfiglio G, Bruzzi P, et al. Risk associated with pregnancy in hypertrophic cardiomyopathy. J Am Coll Cardiol [Internet]. 2002 [Citation 13 Nov 2015]; 40(10): [Approx 13 p.]. Available at: http://content.onlinejacc.org/article.aspx?articleid=1130491

12. Gutiérrez Aliaga Y, Chio Naranjo I, Guerra Chang E, Gutiérrez Aliaga Y, Rodríguez Jorge I. Characterization of pregnant women with heart disease at the Hospital Docente Ginecobstétrico "Ramón González Coro". Medisur [Internet]. 2011 [Cited 4 Sept 2015]; 9(5): [Approx 7 p.]. Available at: http://www.medisur.sld.cu/index.php/medisur/article/view/1713.

13. Labrada Comas YR, Bonet Romero O, Quesada Fondín Mi, Garcés Rojas E, Hernández Díaz N. Anaesthesia for pregnant women with pregnancy-associated cardiomyopathy. CCM [Internet]. 2016 Mar [cited 2016 Sep 22]; 20(1): [Approx 10 p.]. Available from: http://scielo.sld.cu/scielo.php?script=sci_arttext&pid=S1560-43812016000100021&lng=es.

14. Hall ME, Eric M. G, Joey P. G. The heart during pregnancy. Rev Esp Cardiol [Internet]. 2011[Cited 2 Sept 2015]; 64(11): [Approx 6 p.]. Available from: http://www.revespcardiol.org/es/el-corazon-durante-el-embarazo/articulo/90034667/.

15. Casellas M. Cardiopathy and gestation. In. Cabero Roura L, Cararach Ratonera V. XIII intensive continuing education course. Maternal-fetal medicine. Madrid: Grupo Menariri; 2011.p. 79-82.

16. Aguilera Castro F, Díaz P, Calderón JC, Gutiérrez I. Cardiopathy and pregnancy: case series. Rev Colomb Anesthesiol [Internet]. 2011 July [cited 2016 Sep 22]; 39(2): [Approx 8 p.]. Available from:

http://www.scielo.org.co/scielo.php?script=sci_arttext&pid=S0120-33472011000200005&lng=en. http://dx.doi.org/10.5554/rca.v39i2.103.
17. Reinoso R, Alcina Vázquez J, Fernández Pérez M, Luna Alonso MC. Incidence of heart disease during pregnancy in Villa Clara. CorSalud [Internet]. 2012 [cited 20 Jul 2015];4(3):[approx. 4 p.]. Available from: http://www.corsalud.sld.cu/sumario/2012/v4n3a12/embarazo.html

18. Vega Gutiérrez E, Rodríguez Velásquez L, Gálvez Morales V, Sainz Cruz LB, García Guevara C. Incidence and treatment of congenital heart disease in San Miguel del Padrón. Rev Cubana Med Gen Integr [Internet]. 2012 Sep [cited 2016 Sep 22] ; 28(3): [Approx 15 p.]. Available At: http://scielo.sld.cu/scielo.php?script=sci_arttext&pid=S0864-21252012000300002&lng=es
19. Evert Jiménez C, Andrés Zapata-Cárdenas. Enfermedad valvular mitral y embarazo: una amenaza latente Mitral Valve Heart Disease and Pregnancy: A Latent Threat Doença valvular mitral e gravidez: uma ameaça latente. Med U B P [Internet]. 2013 [Cited 12 Sept 2015]; 32(1):[Approx 6 p.]. Available en: http://www.sci.unal.edu.co/scielo.php?script=sci_arttext&pid=S0120-48742013000100005&lng=es&nrm=is.
20. Valladares-Carvajal F, Bernia-Sarría S, González-Rodríguez C. Cardiopathies and pregnancy. Rev Finlay [Internet]. 2011 [cited 2015 Aug 19]; 1(1):[approx. 3 p.]. Available from: http://www.revfinlay.sld.cu/index.php/finlay/article/view/23
21. Acho-Mego Segundo C, Paredes-Salas JR.Considerations on acquired heart disease and gestation. Rev Peru Ginecol Obstet [internet]. 2011 [Cited 12 Nov 2015]; 57(3): [Approx 6 p.]. Available at: http://www.scielo.org.pe/scielo.php?script=sci_arttext&pid=S2304-51322011000300009&lng=en&nrm=iso.

22. Mendoza-Calderón S A, Hernández-Pacheco JA, Estrada-Altamirano Al, Nares-Torices MÁ, Orozco Méndez H, Hernández-Muñoz VA. Initial evaluation of congenital heart disease with short circuit in pregnancy. Perinatol. Reprod. [Internet]. 2012 Sep [cited 2016 Sep 23] ; 26(3) : [Approx 12 p .]. Available from: http://www.scielo.org.mx/scielo.php?script=sci_arttext&pid=S0187-53372012000300007&lng=es.

23. Mayorga HC, Rodríguez AJG, Enríquez GG, Alarcón R, Gamboa W C, Capella SD, et al. Cardiopatías congenital heart disease: diagnosis prenatal diagnosis y follow-up. Rev Chil Obstet Gynecol [Internet]. 2013 Oct [Cited 2016 Sep 23] ; 78(5): [Approx 8 p.]. Available from:

http://www.scielo.cl/scielo.php?script=sci_arttext&pid=S0717-75262013000500004&lng=en.

24. Román Rubio P, Pérez Torga JE, Guerra Chang E, Hernández García S, Gómez Graham DT, Cotilla Morales E. General recommendations for the management of the pregnant woman with heart **disease** (Part I). Rev Cubana Cardiol Cir Cardiovasc [Internet]. 2010 [Cited 12 Jun /2015];16(3): [Approx 8 p.]. Available at: http://**www.bvs.sld.cu/revistas/car/vol16_3_10/car08310.html.**

25. Fayad Saeta Y, López Barroso R, Erasto Lardoeyt Soto, San Pedro López MI. Cardiopathy and pregnancy. Rev Cubana Obstet Ginecol [Internet]. 2009 Dec [cited 2016 Sep 22] ; 35(4): [Approx 11 p.]. Available from: http://scielo.sld.cu/scielo.php?script=sci_arttext&pid=S0138-600X2009000400005&lng=en.

26. González Maqueda I, Armada Romero E, Díaz Recasens J, Gallego García de Vinuesa P, García Moll , Ana González García[a] , et al. Clinical practice guidelines of the Spanish Society of Cardiology in pregnant women with heart disease. Rev Esp Cardiol [internet]. 2000 [cited 24 Sept 2015]; 53(11):[Approx 21 p.].Available from: http://www.revespcardiol.org/es/guias-practica- clinica-sociedad-espanola/articulo/12087/

27. Rodríguez Hidalgo N, Cuité León E, Cordero Isaac R. Cardiopathies and pregnancy. In: Manual de diagnóstico y tratamiento en Obstetricia y Perinatología. Havana: Ecimed; 2000. p. 294- 304.

28. Valdivia E, PA. Doblas, JJ. Sánchez-Rosas, M. A. Barber, I. Eguiluz, JV. Hijano, M. Suárez, JR. Andarica, I. Aguilera and J. Herrera. Mitral stenosis in a pregnant woman. A case report. Clin Invest Gin Obst Gynecol [Internet]. 2003 [Cited 13 Nov 2015[; 30(9): [Approx 4 p.] Available from: http://www.elsevier.es/es-revista-clinica-e-investigacion-ginecologia-obstetricia-7-articulo-articular-mitral-stenosis-gestante-a-proposito-13055012.

29. Alonso Gómez AM, Borrás X, del Castillo, González AE, Mazón P, Monserrat L, et al. ESC clinical practice guideline for the management of cardiovascular disease during the treatment of cardiovascular disease during the first year of life. pregnancy. A critical view from Spanish cardiology Rev Esp Cardiol. 2012;65(2):113- 118.

30. Pijuan Domènecha A, Gatzoulis MA. Pregnancy and heart disease. Rev Esp Cardiol [Internet]. 2006 [Cited 12 Sept 2015]; 59(9): [Approx 14 p.]. Available from: http://www.revespcardiol.org/es/embarazo-cardiopatia/articulo/13092801/

31. Rodríguez Alvárez M, Ojeda González JJ, Álvarez Figueredo Z, Barco Díaz V. Guía de práctica clínica para la asistencia a la paciente obstétrica con cardiopatía: una alternativa de actuación para el anestesiólogo. Medisur [Internet]. 2011 [Cited 10 Oct 2015]; 9(5): [Approx 8 p.]. Available at: http://www.medisur.sld.cu/index.php/medisur/article/view/1805/6579.

32. Braunwald. Contemporaryevaluation and management of hypertrophic cardiomyopathy. Circulation. 2002; 106(21):1312-1316.

33. Thaman R, Varnava A, Hamid MS, Firoozi S, Sachdev B, Condon M, et al. Pregnancy related complications in women with hypertrophic cardiomyopathy. Heart 2009; 89(3):752- 756.

34. Melvin KR, Richarson PJ, Olsen EG, Daly K, Jackson G. Peripartum cardiomyopathy due to myocarditis. N Engl J Med. 2009; 307(7): 731-734.

35. Patton DE, Lee W, Cotton DB, Miller J, Carpenter RJ Jr, Huhta J, et al. Cyanotic maternal heart disease in pregnancy. Obstet Gynecol Surv 2010; 45(8):594-600.

36. Manso B, Gran F, Pijuán A, Giralt G, Ferrer Q, Betrián P, et al. Pregnancy and congenital heart disease. Rev Esp Cardiol. 2008;61(3):236-43

37. Schlemmer M. Pregnancy in patient with congenital heart defect. Wien Klin. Wochenschr. 1995; 107(20):608-12.

38. Acho-Mego SC, Paredes-Salas, José Raúl. Considerations on congenital heart disease and gestation. Rev Peru Ginecol Obstet [Internet]. 2011 [Cited 12 Nov 2015]; 57(3): [Approx 7 p.]. Available at: http://www.scielo.org.pe/scielo.php?script=sci_arttext&pid=S2304-51322011000300008&lng=en&nrm=iso

39. Fayad Saeta Y, López Barroso R, Lardoeyt Soto E, San Pedro López MI. Cardiopathy and pregnancy. Rev Cubana Obstet Ginecol [Internet]. 2009 [cited 3 Aug 2015];35(4):[approx. 5 p.]. Available from: http://bvs.sld.cu/revistas/gin/vol35_4_09/gin05409.htm

40. Emergency Cardiac Care Committee, Subcommittees and Task Forces of the American Heart Association. 2005 American Heart Association Guidelines for Cardiopulmonary Resuscitation and Emergency Cardiac Care. Part 108: Cardiac arrest association with pregrancy. Circulation [Internet]. 2009 [Cited 13 Nov 2015]; 112(4): [Approx 35 p.]. Available from: http://circ.ahajournals.org/content/112/24_suppl

41. Thanajiraprapa T, Phupong V. Pregnancy complications in women with heart disease. J Maternal-Fetal Neonatal Med [Internet]. 2010 [Cited 13 Nov

2015]; 23(10): [Approx 5p]. Available from: http://www.ncbi.nlm.nih.gov/pubmed/19903109.

42. Labrada Comas YR, Bonet Romero O, Quesada Fondín M, Garcés Rojas E, Hernández Díaz N. Anaesthesia for pregnant women with pregnancy-associated cardiomyopathy. ccm [Internet]. 2016 Mar [cited 2016 Sep 23]; 20(1): [Approx 10p.]. Available from: http://scielo.sld.cu/scielo.php?script=sci_arttext&pid=S1560-43812016000100021&lng=es.

43. Gómez Flores JR, Márquez Manlio F. Arrhythmias in pregnancy: How and when to treat? Arch Cardiol Méx [Internet]. 2007 Jun [cited 2016 Sep 23]; 77(Suppl 2): [Approx 8 p]. Available from: http://www.scielo.org.mx/scielo.php?script=sci_arttext&pid=S1405-99402007000600005&lng=es.

44. Yáñez-Gutiérrez L, Cerrud-Sánchez CE, López-Gallegos D, Márquez-González H, García- Pacheco MB, Jiménez-Santos M. Pregnancy in women with congenital heart disease. Cardiol [Internet]. 2015 [Cited 13 Nov 2015]; 26(4): [Approx 7 p.]. Available from: http://www.scielo.org.mx/pdf/rmc/v26n4/v26n4a7.pdf.

45. Suárez D OH, Vargas Acero LR, Valderrama Hernández JA. Epidural anesthesia for cesarean section in Ebstein's anomaly. Rev. colomb. anesthesiol [Internet]. 2011 July [cited 2016 Sep 23].;39(2):[Approx10p.].Availablefrom: http://www.scielo.org.co/scielo.php?script=sci_arttext&pid=S0120-33472011000200008&lng=en. http://dx.doi.org/10.5554/rca.v39i2.101.

46. Ocenes Reinoso R, Alsina Vázquez J, Fernández Pérez M, Luna Alonso MC. Incidence of heart disease during pregnancy in the province of Villa Clara. CorSalud [Internet]. 2012 Jul- Sep [Cited 13 Nov 2015]; 4(3): [Approx 6 p.]. Available at: http://www.corsalud.sld.cu/sumario/2012/v4n3a12/embarazo.html

47. Fayad Saeta Y, López Barroso R, Erasto Lardoeyt Soto, San Pedro López MI. Cardiopathy and pregnancy. Rev Cubana Obstet Ginecol [Internet]. 2009 Dec [cited 2016 Sep 23] ; 35(4):[Approx 11p.] Available at: http://scielo.sld.cu/scielo.php?script=sci_arttext&pid=S0138-600X2009000400005&lng=en.

48. Halla M, Georgeb E, Granger J. The heart during pregnancy. Rev Esp Cardiol [Internet].2011 [Cited 13 Nov 2015]; 64(11): [Approx 6 p.]. Available from: http://www.revespcardiol.org/es/el-corazon-durante-el-embarazo/articulo/90034667/

ANNEXES

Annex 1

Primary data collection model

Name

Address

Age
Gestational age

Probable date of delivery

Diagnosis of heart disease: -before pregnancy
-during pregnancy
Type of heart disease: -rheumatic
-Congenita

-Other

Specific Cardiac Injury:

Did you receive obstetric advice: Yes No

Before pregnancy

During pregnancy

6.-Type of orientation:	For your doctor	By Cardiologist
(a) May impregnate or		
maintaining the pregnancy		
b) Do not impregnate		
c) Termination of pregnancy		
(d) Did not receive counselling		

He presented cardiovascular complications:Yes No

Type of complication: If present, this occurred:

First trimester of pregnancy

Second trimester of pregnancy

Third trimester of pregnancy

Functional capacity: 12 3 4
Pathways of delivery: Euthocic
Caesarean section
Instrumented
If dystocic delivery indicated by: Obstetrics
Cardiology

Birth weight:Full term

Pre-term

Status of the product of Pregnancy: healthy NB
Deceased NB
Dead foetus Other

Annex 2

Informed Consent

Provincial Teaching Hospital "V. I. Lenin" Provincial Teaching Hospital Holguín I approve my participation in a research aimed at the study Clinical-epidemiological characterisation of heart disease in pregnancy. Year 2015. V.I. Lenin Hospital. I am willing to participate in the clinical interview and I allow the use of the information by the researchers.I authorise the use of the results in publications as well as for other research purposes as long as they are beneficial to the development of science. I affirm and confirm that our participation is completely voluntary. I have asked all the questions I considered necessary about the research and in case I would like to provide any new information or receive more information about the study I know I can contact you:

Dr. Erick Ramón Silva Bermúdez

I agree with all of the foregoing and for the record I have hereunto set my hand this day of the year .

Signature of Patient

PatientSignature of Investigator

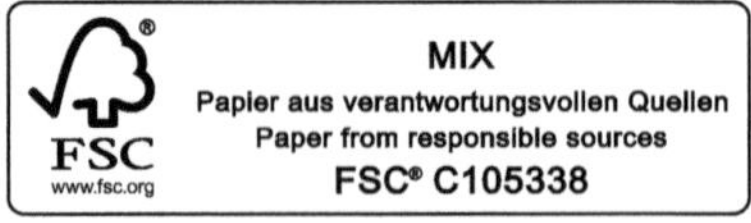

Printed by Books on Demand GmbH, Norderstedt / Germany